# Hope in the Shadows
## --*My Breast Cancer Journey*

***Jeremiah 29:11*** *For I know the plans I have for you, declares The Lord, plans to prosper you and not to harm you, plans to give hope and a future.*

November 2014, Vicki Marney

## Acknowledgements:

To both God and my husband, you were with me and gave me hope, even before I knew I needed it. You walked with me on this journey, and my heart belongs to you. Without your love and encouragement, I am not sure where I would be at this time.

## Dedication:

This work is dedicated to my 5 T's: Thad, Tabitha, Tiffany, Tiara, and Trevor. None of you wanted this path, but your understanding and love helped carry me through. It is my hope that this work will be an inspiration to all of those who have and will conquer cancer. A special place in my heart is reserved for Bobbi Wilson, who was more than a conqueror. Her life and love for God continues to inspire me.

**I am a Breast Cancer Survivor!**

Early in my breast cancer journey, I went to a Breast Cancer Survivor Day event. At the door, they had people sitting at a table, checking everyone in and creating name tags for the attendees. These name tags included how long you were a Survivor--some were 1 year, others 5 years, some 10 years. And amazing to me, some were 20 years and more! I told them I was newly diagnosed, so I didn't qualify for any of those titles. The wonderful woman at the table kindly told me "You are a Survivor from day one of your diagnosis--so how long?" I don't remember how long it had been, but it was not years, it was months. Now, twenty years later and I'm now amazed to be one of those that can say "I am a Twenty Year Survivor" and here is some of my journey along the way.

## Sunday, Nov. 27, 1994--A Perplexing Message

I stayed home from church that day with our oldest teen-age daughter who was going through a rebellious stage and had refused to go to church. Meanwhile, my husband Jon attended and he had an experience entirely unique in his life. Here is what he told me later that day:

During the service, our pastor had requested that those who needed prayer should come forward. At that point, Jon had a strong impression that there was someone that had a serious problem, 'like maybe cancer or something' and needed prayer. The impression was very clear that God knew about the problem and that it was going to be okay. In addition, the message was that God would be with them *THROUGH* the problem, not around it. Then Jon saw what he described as a vision of something like an X-ray, only reversed, with a large, uneven-edged dark splotch. He felt like God wanted him to share it, but there was an equal impression that the person did not know they had a problem. So then, there was an obvious dilemma—if someone did not know they had a problem, how would they know they needed to go forward for prayer? With this apparent contradiction, he did not feel he could say anything—it just did not make sense.

Meanwhile, among those that had come forward was a woman named Lydia. The pastor subsequently told the congregation that Lydia had previously found a lump in her breast and was going in for a biopsy and was requesting prayer that everything would turn out okay. Jon thought, *"Oh, that is who this message was for"*. Yet this impression was so strong and so unusual, he still felt he needed to tell someone. So, he whispered to another of our daughters who was sitting next to him saying, "The weirdest thing just happened..." Then after the service he told the pastor.

After Jon came home, he also told me and expressed his confusion about how strange it was to have a feeling that God had a message for someone, but that the person did not know they needed to hear it. This was a situation that had never happened to either of us before and has never happened since then.

**Earlier that year... January, 1994**

When Jon came home the first workday of 1994, he brought some unwelcome news. He told me he had received a call from his manager saying that the company had decided to close the office in Portland. His manager said, "You should either look for another job, or prepare to move to the Seattle area, to work from this office." Then Jon said something to me that we would remember forever, "This is going to be a very interesting year". We didn't know at that time how true his statement would be...

## Winter to Spring, 1994

After hearing that we were planning a move to the
Seattle area, our oldest son decided he didn't want to move
with us. Instead, he said he would prefer to move with
some friends to Twin Falls, Idaho. His friends had started
an outreach to street kids there and he wanted to join them
in this ministry.

For us, the next several months were spent
commuting from our home in Gladstone, Oregon, to the
office in Renton, Washington. During that time our two
oldest girls stayed with the families of their friends so they
could continue in their school in Gladstone.

Our two younger children, whom I was
homeschooling, "commuted" with us. The
four of us would drive to and from Seattle and stay four
nights in a hotel during the work-week. I homeschooled the
two little ones in the morning, and the three of us went

house hunting in the afternoon. After Jon finished work on Friday we drove back to Oregon to spend the weekend with our two older girls. We continued this pattern for several months.

We were having no success in finding an affordable and appropriate home for our family in the Seattle area. We could not afford to continue making both our house payment while also renting a hotel room each week. So, we decided a temporary solution would be to stay in a tent at an RV park. Yes, we were homeschooling in a tent! This lasted for several weeks. We connected to the power available for RV's, so we did have heat from a space heater and lighting. I have a vivid memory of the four of us huddling together one night as we listened to the rain and wind outside, pounding our tent and praying the tent was staked down well enough to not fall down on us. This was a humbling experience for us.

One pleasant memory during that time was "bunnies". As the calendar was heading into Spring, there were lots of bunnies also living in this 'park'. The kids and I enjoyed watching them hop across our path as we walked to the lodge area where they had an indoor poor. We also frequently enjoyed 'PE time' in that pool.

It was not evident at the time; however, God was in control. We were frustrated that we were not finding a home, yet the Lord knew what was ahead. A few weeks after we started staying in the tent, Jon was laid off from his job. Thankfully, this ended our commuting--leaving us with our home in Gladstone and the girls didn't have to change schools after all. However, this also meant that Jon needed to quickly find a new job so we would have an income for our family.

## A Time to Weep and a Time to Laugh?

After finding out Jon needed to look for a new job, it was impressed on me that we needed a time to rest and regroup as a family. I know it sounds a bit crazy: we had no income, yet we were going to take time off to "take a family vacation".  At that time, I had a daily calendar--the kind that you tear off each page—and when we returned home after finding out Jon needed a new job, the scripture for that day was Ecclesiastes 3:4 "*A time to weep and a time to laugh*".  That seemed a bit strange and I didn't really understand how it applied to our situation--it made more sense when I read further.

### *Ecclesiastes 1-4*

*"There is an appointed time for everything.  And there is a time for every event under heaven ~ A time to give birth, and a time to die; A time to plant, and a time to*

*uproot what is planted. A time to kill, and a time to*

*heal; A time to tear down, and a time to build up.* ***A time to***

***weep, and a time to laugh;*** *A time to mourn, and a time to*

*dance.*

**Romans 8:28**

*"And we know that God causes all things to work*

*together for good to those who love God, to those who are*

*called according to His purpose."*

**Application in my life**

God has appointed times and seasons for

everything. He knows the time for all things in our life,

including the sad times and the times of laughter. Yes, the

times of sadness or 'the winter' can be difficult, but God

knows the Spring is coming and there will be laughter once

again. God is in control. He has a purpose for everything,

whether we understand that reason or not.

**A Time to Weep**

During the time of our commuting, we also had two different tragedies that affected our family. First a woman who attended our church was kidnapped while on her way to a meet a friend for dinner at a local restaurant. She was coaching the cheer-leading team at the private school at our church, and was a wife and mother of two preschoolers. A couple of weeks later, her car was found 30 miles from where she was last seen. A day later her body was found in a field nearby--she had been raped and then strangled. (Note: this woman's murder was not solved until 10 years later. Using DNA evidence, two men were arrested and charged with her death). Since our girls were not attending the school at our church at that time, they didn't know her well, but many of their church friends did. They had never been to a funeral before, so I decided to give them a choice, whether or not to attend, and they chose to attend and I went with them.

Not long afterwards, one of our 'middle' daughter's closest friends committed suicide at age 13. Our family was in shock and it was difficult to even know what to say to our daughter to comfort her. I was then very glad that I had allowed the girls to go to the funeral of someone they did not know well--at least her friend's funeral was not the first funeral she ever attended. Some say that bad things come in three's --I guess the third part of the 'time to weep' was having our family split apart during the time of commuting, followed by Jon losing his job. This was definitely turning into 'an interesting' and difficult year.

## A Time to Laugh

The 'time to laugh' was the product of our choice to take a week to get away as a family at a Christian retreat and conference park. Since it was off-season, we were allowed to stay on a donation basis, and since we had no income, our donation was rather small. They provided all meals at the main lodge and we stayed in a small dorm style room below the lodge. There were no phones or TV's, so we spent our days together as a family, playing board games. We also enjoyed time together on their big tire swing, a big slide, and hiking the nearby paths. This conference center was surrounded by forest and was adjacent to a state park with hiking trails that lead to numerous beautiful waterfalls. This is an area I personally have found to be not only beautiful, but also peaceful and comforting. It is a place where I have found myself going for a few hours or even a short 'overnight retreat with God' in their small 'Prayer Hut' amid the trees..

This provided a time of peaceful reconnection for our family. After months of separation, our family needed this time to come together again without the distractions of life. Amid all the stress we were allowed time to play and laugh.

## Spring and Summer of Change

While Jon was job hunting, we both applied for temporary work with a temporary job agency. This provided a small income to help us until a permanent job could be found. With our reduced income, we qualified for the (then) recently created Oregon Health Plan (OHP).

When we returned from our family retreat, we were informed that due to technicalities, Jon would not receive unemployment compensation for at least six weeks. We immediately applied for welfare and food stamps; however, we didn't qualify because we had a newer vehicle which was valued at more than was allowed in those programs. However, if we had tried to sell it, we would not receive enough to pay off the loan on it. Also, Jon was scheduled to receive the cash-out on his retirement plan, which was counted as an asset which would also disqualify us (even though we would later have to pay a large tax penalty for using this money before retirement).

The Oregon Health Plan ended up being a wonderful blessing. At that time, a family could qualify for six months of coverage based on one qualifying month of low income.

If anyone would have told us that we would go three months without a full time job for Jon, with none of the usual financial benefits, I would have said, "No way!"; however, it was later evident that God provided for our family in several different ways during this time.

**July 1994--A New Job**

In July, Jon found a contract position with a mid-size computer company. It was a full time position, but since it was a contracted position, it did not include company paid medical insurance, but we were still covered by OHP. I continued working for the temporary employment agency for a few weeks; however, transportation soon became an issue, since we only had one vehicle. A few weeks later, I was involved in a minor car accident and received a minor whiplash, and since my temp job involved heavy lifting, I had doctor's orders to end my job, while receiving treatments for my back pain.

**November 1994--End of OHP Coverage**

So then, after a few months with the new job, we knew our health plan coverage (OHP) was going to end soon. I decided to have a complete physical exam while still covered by insurance. During that exam, my primary care physician performed a manual breast exam and no abnormalities were detected. He asked when I last had a mammogram and I told him I had never had one "because my previous doctor did not recommend one until 40, unless it ran in the family". So, my doctor replied, "Well, you're 40 now--you might as well go have a baseline done". Since he had just done a complete physical including the manual exam and had found nothing suspicious--the mammogram was only ordered as a routine preventative test. Little did I know at that time, how timely this decision would be.

## Tuesday, Nov. 29--My First Mammogram

The day arrived for my first mammogram, and I was escorted to a small room for the exam. The young female technician doing the x-rays was kind and gentle and explained everything as she performed the mammogram. So there I was, on the 29th, enjoying a 'smashing' experience'. After checking the films, the technician returned and explained as she taped a 'BB' on a spot on my left breast, that she needed to take some more X-rays. Since this was my first mammogram, although a bit odd, this did not seem suspicious to me.

A little while later, she came back--this time with a radiologist who placed a film from the mammogram on a lighted screen. He told me they had found a suspicious spot and asked if he could examine me. After he examined me, glancing at the mammogram film on the lighted screen for guidance, he showed me where to feel for a lump and helped me find what the mammogram had detected. I didn't immediately feel anything--it was not close to the surface. But, once I did, I realized I had a lump nearly the size of a walnut! The radiologist advised me to have a biopsy done right away.

"But my insurance is ending at the end of the month!" I was beginning to feel a bit of panic.

"Well then, we better get it done before the end of the month", he said rather matter-of-factly.

I didn't realize at that point that the end of the month was the next day! I contacted Jon, and I spent the rest of the afternoon at a surgeon's office and then having pre-op X-rays. They ordered a full set of blood work done, and they had me in surgery the next afternoon. I was feeling very overwhelmed doing all of this alone with only a phone call to my husband alerting him of what was going on, so he could arrange to go with me to the

hospital for my surgery the next day.

## A Lump in my Throat and Another in my Breast

November 30, 1994, the morning of my surgery was

our ladies' Bible Study, so I was able to attend before going

to the hospital. I was feeling very nervous because I had

never been in the hospital for anything except the birth of

my first child—the other four had been home births. The

ladies at the Bible study prayed over me before I went to

the hospital, which helped to calm my nerves a bit. One of

the ladies prayed that it would turn out to be nothing, but

all along, both Jon and I felt this was going to be one of

those times that God was going to 'carry us through' NOT

'remove' or 'help us around'.

After my surgery, Jon and a family friend were

waiting for me to wake from the anesthesia. Jon told me

what my surgeon had said, "I have been doing this for a long time, and you get so you can recognize when it is cancer, and this one looks pretty suspicious. Of course we will have to wait for the biopsy to come back, but I am pretty sure this is cancer." After Jon told me this, I said, "Jon! That message to you at church was not for Lydia, it was for me! Lydia didn't have cancer, but I DO! The message was for us!"

Because of the message that God had given to Jon for us, I never experienced the 'Why me?' or, 'Oh no—I'm going die!'. Instead, for us, our reaction was, "Oh no! We don't have any insurance anymore—how are we going to pay for this?" God had already told us that He knew, before we even imagined there was a problem. He had told us that it was going to be okay—we just had to trust Him. My thoughts were occupied with "Oh dear, is this going to involve a lot of pain and vomiting?' I'm a wimp when it comes to pain and I hate vomiting and, 'What am I going to have to go through—to get to the 'other side' of this—to get to being okay again?' We had a year ahead of us to learn to trust God fully.

## The Big C

During the first week after surgery, I had a return visit with my surgeon for a post-op visit. The biopsy confirmed that I did have cancer--the big C! The cancer went to the 'surgical ' (where they removed the tumor during the biopsy surgery) and they needed to go back and take a little more. This could mean a possible mastectomy--removing the entire breast--"just to make sure they got it all". I had a 'hormone positive' cancer which was very aggressive, meaning we needed to proceed quickly. My surgeon presented the possible options going forward. He told me to begin by going back to my primary physician and get referrals for an oncologist and a radiologist.

**Early December, 1994**

When I went to see my primary doctor, he was apologetic that he had not found the tumor during my exam. I assured him that even after being shown where to feel, it was difficult to detect, and I felt no blame was deserved. Since my doctor was a Christian, I shared with him the special message that God had given to Jon, and told him it was all in God's timing. If he had not sent me for the baseline mammogram, my cancer probably would have not been found before it got to a much later stage. I thanked him and waited as his office staff called to schedule appointments for me with an oncologist and a radiologist,

Everyone at the hospital was so kind and caring towards me. My doctor's nurse (who happened to also be my doctor's wife) handed us the names and addresses for my new doctors, along with appointment times. She also told us that it is very common for cancer patients to become very attached to their oncologist. She also mentioned that Dr. N (the oncologist) was 'different' and he would either drive us nuts or we would love him. We chuckled somewhat nervously and wondered what she meant...

## Contacting Family with the News

Our oldest son was living in Twin Falls, Idaho at the time, with other college-age friends. They didn't have a working phone or cell phones, so it took us about a week before we were able to reach him. When we did reach him later by phone and I told him of my diagnosis, he responded with, "Whoa!  When did this happen?"

I told him the mammogram was done on Nov. 29th and he said "Oh, my gosh!  I was at a prayer service that day, and I suddenly felt an urge to pray for you!"  Not only was I surprised that my 19 year old son was praying at the same time that I needed prayer, but that he was *listening.* Thank you Lord for small blessings.

My father had been retired for several years and my parents had been living the life of 'snowbirds', in Yuma, Arizona for about six months of the year. They had already left for the winter, so I had to call to tell them of my diagnosis. After hearing my news, my mother said to me, "Well, you know your Aunt Earlene and Aunt Betty had breast cancer a couple years ago--they both had mastectomy's". (Note: They never had any further treatments following their mastectomies, since it was thought that if you had a mastectomy, the cancer

was removed, leaving no need for further treatment.)

"Actually mom, no, I didn't know that", I replied.

Both of these aunts lived in California, so we did

not see them very often, and it was just simply not

something we talked about. In other words, breast cancer

DID run in my family. My mom's father had died of

stomach cancer years before, and then, a few months after

my diagnosis, another of my mother's sisters was diagnosed

with cancer, but it was throat cancer from being a heavy

smoker. My family has been highly affected from cancer--

Both aunts had reoccurrences awhile after my diagnosis

and all of these family members eventually died from the

disease.

**Thoughts About My Diagnosis**

The next few days and weeks were kind of a blur to me. I had always been so healthy--I rarely even got the flu and almost never took medications. In fact, I also had never used sugar substitutes, rarely drank soda, and never smoked--many of the typical things that are commonly blamed for cancer. Most doctor visits had been for my kids and the only visits to the ER were from my children's occasional bumps and scrapes. Stitches here, a sprain there--but always the kids and always minor.

Yes, my husband needed knee surgery back in 1981. Then he had his gall bladder out in 1992, and a burst appendix following a car accident. But the only time I had been the patient in a hospital was in 1975, when I gave birth to our first child. So then, in 1994, this was all new to me, and I had trouble grasping the idea that I actually had a life threatening illness. I would be seeing multiple doctors and these doctors would be prodding, poking, and performing lots of tests and more blood work than I ever imagined; sometimes every day!

At night, my husband and I laid next to each other and talked about the possibilities ahead of us, and even though we felt the assurance that it was all in God's hands, it was still scary and, at times, overwhelming. After being told that the size of my tumor put me between stage 1 and stage 2, and with the aggressiveness, we were assuming that I would need a mastectomy. Jon assured me that he would be with me through it all, and that I would still be the beautiful woman he had married. But how was I going to feel about losing my breast? Even though Jon was saying that it wouldn't change his feelings about me, how would I feel about myself? That was a concern that Jon had for me, too. He didn't want me to feel like I was any less of a woman. He was my rock and support during this time (after God, of course).

As much as everyone says that it shouldn't make a difference, a woman's breasts and her hair are still a huge part of her femininity and I was looking at the possibility of losing both. Those are a real and important part of being a woman. We held each other close and cried together as we grieved a part of my femininity going away.

I may have been strong on the outside, but on the inside I was a crumbling, emotional mess--with tears quickly and sometimes unexpectedly showing up. I was just able to keep most of those times in private, usually at night in our bedroom.

## Our Research

With my husband being a major computer guy, once we found out I had breast cancer, it was only natural for us to immediately get online and began to look up everything we could find about breast cancer. Although this was before the spread of the 'Internet' and 'Google' made searches easy, we were able to look up online support, the Komen Foundation, common treatments and what to expect.

If it had to do with BC we probably looked it up. We actually found this helpful when we began meeting my new doctors--my new 'Cancer Team'. We also found many online support groups as well as blogs being kept by other cancer patients. This all gave me added comfort regarding my situation.

**Doctors and More Doctors!**

As I noted before, the week after the biopsy was filled with doctor visits. After returning to my primary doctor, I had more post op visits with my surgeon, and then met with my new radiologist, and my new oncologist. Then, it was back to the surgeon again--appointments every day that week.

**Meeting my Radiologist**

My first appointment with a cancer doctor was with my radiologist. He showed us all the statistics for various breast cancer treatment plans. Those without any treatment, the statistics after a lumpectomy followed by radiation, and also after a mastectomy (which would not require radiation because the tissue is ALL removed). He said that the statistics for a lumpectomy followed by radiation were virtually the same as someone who had a mastectomy. He also said he thought that a woman of my age would probably choose to save the breast, if that was an option, and if the statistics showed it was a reasonable choice. Of course, we were very happy to hear that it would be OUR choice whether to have a mastectomy or a lumpectomy-- maybe there was a chance of saving my breast. Some women are not given this choice, even though it should be theirs to make.

Overall, when facing medical decisions, this should be a defining criterion: *Give people the facts and statistics and allow them to make their own choice, please--their body, their choice*!

Then the radiologist shared a personal opinion about these options. He said that there are a percentage of women who have received a cancer diagnosis who will still have a reoccurrence, even after either of these choices. (If I remember correctly, I believe it was about 5%). In his opinion, if a woman chooses a mastectomy and was in the percentage that had a reoccurrence, there would then be no remaining breast tissue. In that case, the reoccurrence would likely go into the bones, making treatment more difficult. However, if the woman had chosen a lumpectomy, there would still be remaining tissue and she could then have a mastectomy to remove the remaining breast tissue, and, hopefully, all of the cancer. This explanation made sense to me, so we chose to have the surgeon remove a little more tissue and the nearby 'lymph nodes' during the second surgery (hoping to get any remaining cancer), rather than a mastectomy.

## Meeting Mr. Rogers?

Before meeting my oncologist, Jon and I were talking outside his office. Jon asked, "I wonder what kind of person would choose oncology as a specialty--it seems like it would be a difficult profession, spending so much time with so many terminally ill patients". We found out when we met Dr. N (my oncologist). As he walked into the room, he greeted us with a big smile and with a lilt in his voice, asking "And how are we today?" We looked at each other with a slight grin, but said nothing. He had the same tone of voice and perkiness of Mr. Rogers--yes, Mr. Rogers, as in the children's TV program!

At one point, a nurse came in to tell him he had an urgent phone call, so he had to step out of the exam room for a moment. As soon as he stepped out, we both burst into laughter. "I guess we found out what type of person would choose oncology as their specialty..." Our nervousness about meeting with Dr. N had been lessened. And in case you are wondering, we both loved Dr. N...

When he returned, Dr. N went through all the statistics with us, just as my radiologist had. When I told Dr. N what the radiologist had said about reoccurrence, Dr. N didn't seem too happy that the radiologist had told us his opinion—he goes with statistics, not opinion. However, he did not try to convince us to change our minds. He told us that due to the size of my tumor and the aggressiveness, I would need to follow up with six months of chemotherapy, but the outcome of my second surgery would determine how aggressive the chemo would be. They would also remove lymph nodes during this second surgery to determine if any lymph tested positive for cancer. That information would determine which type of chemo I should have--if there was any lymph node involvement, it would mean a more aggressive type of chemo.

## Insurance Coverage

As far as the insurance and payments went, we were originally on the new Oregon Health Plan (OHP). Since Jon had lost his job and went without a job for about three months--OHP was the only assistance we actually qualified for at the time. Some of the rules about receiving assistance did not seem very intelligent for some programs, but for the OHP, our coverage was good for six months. However, the six months were up at the end of November and we had not reapplied. Jon had been hired as a contract employee for a new job in July, and we were making too much money to re-qualify. However, as a contractor, Jon did not have any employer provided insurance--and we were facing the possibility of huge medical bills.

We found ourselves spending long hours on the phone, trying to determine our options. We discovered a very helpful state senator who had supported the adoption of OHP, and whose wife was also going through BC treatments. (Later, we were saddened by the news that she had died from breast cancer). We followed his advice, which was "Do whatever you need to do, to make sure you don't fall through the cracks". We were told that since Jon was an independent contractor and was not on a salary, he could reduce his schedule to only work the number of days that would still keep us qualified for OHP. Basically, that meant his earnings had to stay below what was considered poverty level. I was also told to have my doctor write a note saying that I had been diagnosed with a life-threatening illness. The note also specified that I would require care which could be provided by my husband. This would provide an appropriate reason for him to miss work--

and the note also requested immediate re-

instatement of our OHP coverage, without break, so that

any and all medical care would be covered.

*Note: At that time, you only had to qualify during*

*the month you applied and then if approved, the coverage*

*was good for six months. Even if during the following*

*month, you got a wonderful job that paid really well, or you*

*won a lottery, you were still eligible for six months. So, all*

*he had to do for approval was make sure he didn't work*

*any more days than would still qualify during the month of*

*application. This is no longer the case--only women,*

*babies, and sometimes seriously ill adults with a low*

*income qualify, and I believe there is a three month income*

*qualification period now.*

The rules in 1994 meant that Jon was able to stay

home from work on the days of my appointments--and

there were a LOT of them during that December. He was

able to be with me for all those discussions with the doctors about treatments. This was important, since my brain was still in 'shock', and he was also able to be there for all the 'firsts'. This was very helpful and appreciated by me. On the other hand it meant we had a lean Christmas that year.

*Note: I think it is important for anyone who is receiving information concerning a serious health issue to ALWAYS have someone with you during appointments. When receiving this type of information, it is very common for your brain to be in such shock and stress, that you are likely to have difficulty understanding, comprehending, and remembering what is being told to you.*

## Back on OHP

The other great thing about being placed back onto OHP was that we had ZERO co-pay! Jon's company offered to put him on as a salaried employee so he would qualify for the company insurance; however, he declined the offer, because he assumed the insurance company would consider it to be a pre-existing condition. This usually meant the insurance would put a very low ceiling on what they would cover for ANY cancer treatments. In addition, we would probably have to pay a percentage of all bills as a co-pay. This would have added up to a significant amount, and set us back financially even more than the limited work hours and other miscellaneous expenses.

## Dec. 16, 1994--Surgery #2

I chose to have the second surgery done early in December, because I didn't want it too near to Christmas, plus I was anxious to "get any remaining cancer out of my body". They were also planning to remove a 'patch' of lymph nodes from my armpit to check for any positive lymph nodes and I requested to have a *Groshong Catheter (a port that leads directly to the main artery) installed during the surgery for later use during chemo.

*Note: After telling our church family about my cancer diagnosis, our Pastor's wife introduced me to 'Judy', her Mary Kay Consultant. Judy had gone through breast cancer about a year or so before me and our diagnosis and treatments were very similar. Judy was a great help, in that she shared some of the things to expect, and she also told me about using a 'port'. (Mine was called a Groshong Catheter). Although she ended up needing to have hers *removed early because of infection, she said she*

*appreciated it so much. With it, all blood draws and*

*infusions could be done through the 'port', rather than*

*getting 'poked' each time you have a chemo treatment or*

*need blood drawn. I soon found out that there would have*

*been a LOT of pokes! Thanks for the suggestion, Judy!*

**The Plan**

The surgery went without any problems--the results

from the biopsy in this second surgery determined there

was no further cancer in the breast, but one lymph node

tested positive. That bumped me up to full-fledged Stage 2

Breast Cancer. I would need six 28 day cycles of

aggressive chemo, followed by 6 weeks of radiation (5 days

a week), and then 5 years of hormone therapy on

Tamoxifen. This was "The Plan". Later, three daily

injections--beginning a certain number of days into the

chemo cycle--were added to this 'plan' to help

prevent my white cell counts from dropping too low.

*Note: Prior to the surgery, Jon had the strong impression*

*that there would be ONE positive lymph node--no more and*

*no less--only ONE! And that is exactly what there was--one*

*positive lymph node. Was God walking along with us on*

*this or what? And the Groshong was now in place and*

*ready to serve me well for the next year.*

**Christmas Eve, 1994**

I was recovering from the second surgery well, but

then I noticed redness at the surgery site where they had

removed the lymph nodes (in my armpit). It itched

tremendously! I called my doctor, and was told to go to the

ER--what a way to spend Christmas Eve. It turned out to be

no problem--I actually had an allergic reaction to the tape

used for the bandage. The adhesive mixed with my normal

arm perspiration created a rash. I was instructed to no longer use the typical tape, but to switch to paper tape and given a cream to relieve the itching.

## God's Promise for me

During all this time, I clung to the promise that God had given us: "Everything was going to be okay--*He had it under control,* and *He knew about it before we even had an inkling that there was a problem".* Not to say that I was not still scared or that I wasn't a basket case during those days and weeks. My husband and I would both hold each other at night and frequently cry ourselves to sleep, and we had many restless nights.

When they told me I should have an entire body scan to rule out any other possible cancer, I thought, *"Oh no! Do they think I have cancer somewhere else too?"* I soon found out that this was a routine test for all cancer patients. The night before this scan, I was on the phone with the hospital staff receiving instructions for the scan the next day, when there was a knock on the door. A beautiful bouquet of flowers in a cobalt blue vase was delivered, sent by my husband's office, and someone brought them into the kitchen where I was sitting. I burst into tears, and said, "They're so beautiful!" I found myself apologizing to the person on the phone as I was blubbering. Obviously, all the stress of everything had just overcome me--I am not normally the kind of person who cries over a bouquet of flowers.

From that point on, my life changed so very drastically! I had been a woman who had been very healthy and rarely saw a doctor for myself, or even took aspirin. I now had to start carrying a small calendar to keep track of all my appointments with multiple doctors on a weekly and sometimes daily basis, and taking multiple medications. I was now a "chemo patient"--later to become a

"radiation patient"--something I had never imagined.

## Chemotherapy Treatment Plan

My chemo infusion regimen occurred on day one

and again on day seven of a 28 day cycle. Each treatment

included the following: Zofran, (a very effective anti-

nausea), to be followed by three chemo drugs including

Cytoxan, Adriamycin, and Fluorouracil, (aka 5-FU), and

then a second dose of Zofran. It ALWAYS began and

ended with Zofran. Then, I was sent home with Zofran in

pill form to take for the next couple days. Then, I spent the

rest of the 28 day cycle recovering from these poisons, and

getting frequent blood draws to check my blood counts to

make sure my body was ready for the next 28 day cycle. I

was pleasantly surprised at how well my body tolerated

these drugs. It is still amazing to me how well our medical

staff was able to determine just how much of these chemicals to use to successfully kill off the cancer cells, yet not kill our bodies. I feel God has blessed our minds to be able to do the research needed to be able to accomplish such wonderful results.

*Note: A daily injection for three successive days was added after my first couple treatments, in order to bring up my white cell counts. I never had to have my chemo treatments delayed for low blood counts after the addition of this drug.*

### First Chemo--New Years Day, 1995

My first chemo treatment was done on New Year's day! 1994 had indeed been an 'interesting' year. Now I was starting 1995 with chemotherapy. I went into the oncologist's office and was seated in one of several recliner chairs. They were in a row with IV posts positioned next to each chair along with a small table to place a drink, book, or other personal items. I don't really remember anything about the other patients receiving chemo at the same time, because I was too distracted by what was happening to me. Jon came with me and sat in an extra chair brought in for him.

A nurse explained everything to me, and the order it would occur. The nurse also told me that if I needed to get up for any reason while my infusions were taking place (like using the bathroom) that I needed to do so before they started the Adriamycin, because, "you need to stay still while it is being administered because it could burn you if it escaped your veins". At this point, I told her that I had a Groshong Catheter (which was connected directly to a main artery) and she said, "Oh, good! Then there is no problem!" --another reason for me to be happy that I asked for the Groshong to be inserted!

## A Welcome Surprise

Everything went smoothly, and we returned home to discover some of my Christian friends had come over and cleaned our entire house while I was having my chemo! And they came over during EVERY chemo to do the same--what a blessing! They had also arranged with the ladies of our church and some who were friends that attended other churches, to provide dinners for our family of 7 every night for a while. This was a definite blessing for me, to not have to worry about "What's for dinner?" However, I did learn later that my children did not appreciate it as much. They were very happy when dinners became "normal" again.

*Note: When providing meals for a family in need (especially if there are children in the family, ask if there are specific likes and dislikes in the family. We appreciated ALL the yummy meals that we received from friends;*

*however, fried chicken and casseroles begin to all*

*taste the same after a while.  ;-)*

After I got home from my first treatment and settled into my bed, I watched TV and waited--*waited for what-- you might ask?* Am I going to get sick? The first and last drug in my IV was the anti-nausea medication, Zofran, along with a constant glucose drip during the entire infusion. Then, as I noted before, they sent me home with the same anti-nausea in pill form to take after I got home, with the suggestion that I take them even if I was feeling okay. They made it very clear that it is easier to control nausea before it is a problem than to wait and then try to get it under control--so that is what I did. Remember, I said I don't like vomiting.

I was very fortunate that during that day and the next several days, I felt slightly yucky—rather like having morning sickness; however, I never got sick enough to vomit! The Zofran worked GREAT for me.

However, that first night, I laid in bed, WIDE AWAKE! I couldn't go to sleep! I watched TV, and hoped and prayed I was not keeping Jon awake, because he had to go to work the next day. I didn't fall asleep until about 4 or 5 AM.

When I got to the doctor's office the next morning for them to check my blood (yes, the first of many of those blood draws to check my blood levels), I told my doctor about not being able to sleep, and asked if it could be a side-effect of the chemo.

Dr. N said, "Oh! Didn't I give you a prescription for a mild sleeping pill?"

"No, doctor, you did not".

This was one of many times when we observed that Dr. N probably had ADHD. However, it was very obvious that he was taking steps to be sure he would not miss anything if he was distracted. He had his office provide check lists of each patient's information and their medications, especially chemo drugs. He constantly reviewed the lists and he went over this information several times to make sure everything was correct. He made sure this did NOT affect any of his patients. Yes, as my primary doctor's wife/nurse had told me at the beginning, we learned to love my oncologist--I had the best.

## Kicking the Bucket

The next day, I received a call from Dr. N's office saying that I needed to come in. My white cells had dropped too low and Dr. N wanted to discuss the options. At the office, Dr. N told me that he would be reducing the chemo drugs slightly and that I would need to receive daily injections for three days, beginning a certain number of days into each chemo cycle to help rebuild the

white cells. In the meantime, I needed to stay away from

anyone who was sick because I had no immunity at this

point.

I told him, "There is one problem with that, Dr. N--

I just got a call to go pick up my six year old son from

school, because he has the flu!"

Dr. N said, "Then you will just have to stay away

from him--you can NOT care for him!"

So, guess who got to take care of a sick son? Yes, my

husband, who is VERY sensitive to smells! After I got

home from my appointment and picking up our six year

old, I had settled our son on the sofa in the lower level of

our tri-level home, with the TV on children's programs and

a bowl for 'the results of the flu' while I went into the

kitchen to watch TV there. When Jon got home, he went

downstairs to check up on our son. Not knowing I had

placed the bowl on the floor next to Trevor, Jon "kicked the bucket". OK, it was a bowl, but bucket sounds more dramatic... Jon came up to tell me what happened and grabbed a large bunch of paper towels.

The next several minutes, (which I know seemed more like hours to Jon), he spent with a towel covering his nose and mouth, as he went back and forth between getting more paper towels from the kitchen, and going back down to "clean up". Each time he would look at me with eyes that seemed to say, "Do I really have to do this? I'm going to add to the mess...", yet knowing he could not ask me to do it--he was the only one who could "do the nasty job". I think he had a renewed appreciation that this was usually a 'Mom job'.

At one point, after making several trips, I asked him, "How much was there?" And he responded with, "I don't know, but it's a LOT!" I will say though, I had to work hard not to chuckle, because I know it was difficult for him, but it DID provide me with a little humor--poor guy.

## A Change of Scenery

After my first chemo treatment, Dr. N received notification from the Oregon Health Plan that I could no longer receive my treatments in the clinic. Instead, I had to have them as an inpatient at a hospital. This meant the rest of my treatments were done as requested by OHP, as an inpatient at a small local hospital.

Each time, I would check in through the emergency room, be assigned a room, put into a hospital gown, and received my treatments there. I also went to the ER to get my injections to build my white cell count, so the ER staff got to know me on a first name basis. I didn't even have to tell them who I was or what I needed, because they had

already received my doctor's orders. We made the
comment at the time that it was strange and somewhat
unsettling to be on a first name basis with an ER staff...

## Losing My Hair

Hair loss during chemo is dependent on numerous
factors including what drugs you are given, the timing of
the treatments, and the dosage strength. Adriamycin
usually causes complete hair loss about three weeks
following the first treatment. When I say 'complete hair
loss', I mean that you lose your hair EVERYWHERE!
That included eyelashes, eyebrows, underarm, legs, and
yes, even pubic hair. I was fortunate that I did not lose my
eyelashes or eyebrows, but everywhere else? Yep! I will
say that having hairless under arms and legs was something
of a blessing--no shaving necessary--and those places were

the last to grow new hair. I referred to that as a benefit of chemo, rather than a negative...

I was told by Dr. N that on day number 21, my hair brush would begin to find more and more hair in it, and within another day or so it would just begin dropping freely with every movement of my head. He was right--to the day! It was surprising to me how fast it happened. Some of the same friends who were involved with cleaning my house and providing meals, began gathering donations toward purchasing a wig for me.

**Breaking Bald**

One of the women who often checked me in at the hospital had beautiful long hair. Since I was now bald, I silently admired her hair and hoped that she appreciated the ability to have such beautiful long hair, and hoped that someday, mine would again be long.

Another day, my oldest daughter's boyfriend arrived at the door to pick her up for a date--with all his hair shaved off! No, he had not done it in honor of me--he just thought it would be cool. I was in shock--how could someone who had great hair, just CHOOSE to shave it all off? He obviously did not understand the thoughts of a bald cancer patient...

## Pushing my Envelope--A Redhead?

Right after I lost my hair, I had the opportunity to attend an event at a local hospital for cancer patients and hospital professionals who worked with cancer patients. It was sponsored by a business that provided wigs, hats, and head wraps, primarily for women who had lost their hair from cancer or Alopecia.

It turned out that all of the other attendees were either hospital professionals or women whose hair had grown back. I was the only one there who didn't

have hair! So, guess who was asked to be a 'model' for all

the wigs, hats, and head wraps? I was very newly bald and

very self-conscious, but with no other options, I felt

compelled to assist. Afterwards, I was quite happy that they

had 'pushed my envelope'. I was a brunette, a blonde and

yes, even a redhead. I had straight hair, curly hair, short

hair, long hair, and everything in between. Being a natural

brunette, usually with a shoulder length bob or long hair, I

was quite surprised when everyone in attendance thought I

looked best as a short-haired redhead!

**In Search of a Wig**

I first began my search for a wig at the american

cancer Society. They have wigs that have been donated

(usually previously worn by other cancer patients). I did

find a wig there, however, it just did not look like me.

Most of their wigs were more full than I had worn

my hair (I had a medium length bob, that curled under at

the ends). I took the wig; however, my friends decided to

begin a fund to buy a wig that would suit me better.

I began the second part of my search by going to a

hair salon where a friend was working (one of the gals who

had donated money towards the new wig).. She tried

several wigs on me and later told me that she was shocked

at how freely my hair was falling out--she was afraid to

touch it. Even her softest touch caused more hair to fall. I

had begun to save each handful as it fell (while at home) in

a small bag. I think that bag is still somewhere in my

garage (isn't everything?).

At first, I was trying to be very gentle with it by not

scrubbing like I used to do. However, within a few days, it

was clear it was not helping much, so I made an

appointment at a large wig store in Portland for the

following Saturday. The morning of my appointment, I decided to scrub my head thoroughly while taking my shower and it felt so good. But when I was finished, there was not much hair left, so I wrapped a bandana over my head to go to the wig store.

When I got to the wig store, they tried on many styles, but most of them were too fluffy and/or thick and they just did not fit my style--I was not a big fluffy style gal. Eventually they found one that was pretty much like my 'old hair' except no grey and had a reddish highlight.  I LOVED it! In fact, I said that if my new hair didn't come back the same color*, I was going to dye it...which I did and now still do.

*Note:  When a cancer patient's hair grows back, it is possible it will come back a different color.  I met a lady in a support group who had a couple reoccurrences, and had to go through chemo again, each time--losing her hair.

*Each time her hair grew back, it was a different*

*color! I think she eventually ended up with snowy white.*

## Reactions to My Wig

The following morning at church was my first outward display of my new wig, and it was such a good match that people did not realize I was wearing a wig! One older, special lady friend of mine gave me a big hug during the greeting time, and I felt the wig slide slightly. I feared it might fall, and warned her. She was very surprised that it was a wig. After I told the Pastor's wife, she said, "I could tell there was something different, but I wouldn't have guessed it was a wig! I just thought maybe you had gone and had your hair styled and colored, just to feel better!"

That made me feel better about the wig, but I still felt self-conscious about it, often fearing it might fall off or something. I also found that even though a wig covers everything, it still doesn't go down quite as far in the back, as your natural hair line does and it feels a bit drafty.

The following weekend, we went to an Oregon Assembly of God Marriage Encounter weekend (we had been involved as helpers for several years) and we had decided we wanted to shave off the remaining hair that weekend. My remaining hair was so sparse that it just made me look sickly, but Jon forgot to bring his electric shaver with him. We were afraid to use a razor on me, because he was afraid of cutting me. We decided to go next door to Walmart and buy some Nair!

Yes, I said Nair--as Jon put it I had a "Nair shampoo"! My smooth bald head looked so much better and I looked healthier, but I was still self-conscious my appearance. I was also worried about the wig blowing off while at the beach, especially when we walked across an elevated bridge multiple times while we were helping transport luggage into the hotel. It was very windy, which is typical at the Oregon Coast, and I imagined my wig blowing off my head and across the parkway below-- and at that point I was not finding that to be humorous!

One thing that I regret is that because I was so shy about my bald head, I didn't have any photos taken of me bald, and I only have a couple with my hair real short. In fact, I don't even have any photos of me wearing the wig! As my 20 year Anniversary draws near, I wish that I could have created some scrapbook pages to display at my party, but I don't have any photos to scrapbook. That makes me sad now.

**All the Support You Can Get**

When I first was told I had cancer, I knew that I wanted to meet with a support group. Somewhere there were others who also had cancer. And hopefully somewhere with other women who had 'made it through the battles' and could help arm me for my own battle. I didn't realize at the time that I would end up deciding on three different groups to try. I ended up deciding on two that I continued with through my journey.

## Hospital Support Group

I started with a Breast Cancer Support Group at the hospital across the street from my oncologist. We met once a week and we were in various stages of our treatments. It was led by two cancer nurses at the hospital and each session covered different parts of the journey. We each shared a bit of our own story and it was such a relief to meet women who were going through, or had already gone through, many of the same issues that I was facing.

Some had chosen mastectomies, some lumpectomy's, and some were never given a choice. Most had gone through--or were currently going through--chemo and some had radiation therapy. Many were older women who were past menopause and very few were my age or younger. Some had positive hormone responsive cancer and were put on Tamoxifen. We talked about getting sick from chemo, side effects from various treatments, and everything else we had in common and what was different.

We talked about insurance coverage, discrimination towards cancer patients, and how to deal with some of the side effects, such as hot flashes (chemo often puts women into premature menopause). There was one older woman in the group who threw in a question about hot flashes. She said, "What I want to know is when do we run out of hot flashes?" We all burst into laughter.

Another day, this same older woman also told us about how she had gotten the flu (not from chemo) and when she vomited, her teeth fell into the toilet. Before she knew what had happened, she flushed them down the toilet and now she was waiting for a new set of teeth. Yes, we laughed together and sometimes we cried together.

I found this group to be very helpful to me--so great to find a group of women whom I had so much in common with.

## Christian Support Group

I also found a support group that was for ALL cancer patients--breast, uterine, prostate, brain--you name it, and they were free to join our group. It was also open to the patient's support people--their spouses, or whoever their support person was.

This group was led by a woman who had breast cancer several years before; however, she had a mastectomy, so at that time, they determined she didn't need any further treatment. The other person co-leading the group was a man named Jim who had lost his wife after a long battle with uterine cancer. He was also a male nurse and between the treatments he went to with his wife, and his relationships with the medical staff where he worked, he was able to answer many of our medical questions. *(Note: Later this couple married each other. Judy eventually had a reoccurrence and died from metastatic breast cancer.)*

We began the session each week with discussing how everyone was doing. On my first visit, it turned out that nobody else showed up, so I was able to ask questions and share my questions--all focused on me. This was just before going in for the full body scan, so Jim was able to

assure me that it was a common procedure and did
not mean they thought I might have more cancer. They just
want to check everything out, so they would know best
how to proceed.

Within this group, we had a World War II Fighter
pilot who was now fighting prostate cancer which had
spread throughout his body. He was told his cancer was
terminal and he told them that he was not going to 'pull into
the terminal' until his God told him He was ready for him.

There was a beautiful white-haired woman in a
wheel chair, who was always accompanied by her adoring
husband. She was told that she had terminal brain cancer
and that she only had 6 months to live-and that was 6
YEARS before--and she was now cancer free!  Several
years later, she died--of heart failure!

Another man who was attending was very special—
he delivered 'Singing Telegrams' and was a professional

clown and puppeteer. He enjoyed 'throwing his voice', and he ALWAYS had a joke to start us out (usually pretty corny) and a scripture.

This group met in a room at a large church, and I heard that there had been many 'church people' who questioned whether this was a cancer support group. After all, *"There's an awful lot of laughing going on in there..."*

## A Chemo Patient

Once my chemo treatments were switched to Outpatient at the hospital, I began a 'new normal'. The regimen was: go to the oncologist office and have blood drawn to make sure my counts were high enough for the next treatment. Pick up Dr. N's 'orders' to take with me to the hospital (they also FAXed copies to the hospital). Then, check into outpatient the next day, be escorted to 'my room' where I quickly changed into a hospital gown, and

'get settled in my bed'.

My new friend Judy, a fellow Survivor, came with

me to most of my treatments after Jon had to return to

work. We talked and sometimes played card games during

my infusions.  It was almost like going for a spa treatment,

except I was wearing a hospital gown instead of a spa robe.

I was even brought a menu to choose my lunch, and since it

was the same day of the week each time, the choices were

always the same, so I always chose the quiche. (I'm a

creature of habit. Ha Ha).

That was fine until my final treatment at the

hospital, before I switched to Kaiser Health Plan. I ordered

my usual quiche, but after I took the first few bites, all of a

sudden, I felt rather sick. Evidently, my body had decided

that quiche meant I would then be filled with poisons and it had enough! I was unable to eat quiche again for many years. Too bad, since I liked quiche...

When I returned home after each treatment, I would come home to a clean and fresh smelling house, since my friends always cleaned it while I was having my treatments. Jon had returned to his job, so when I got home, the house was all quiet--too quiet. I really appreciated the love and concern by my friends, by cleaning my house, but I was lonely. I wished they had stayed 'just to chat'. Yet, I never told anyone that was how I was feeling, so it was not really their fault, because they didn't know that was how I was feeling.

The anti-nausea medication was working very well, so I didn't really feel sick, just tired. But how much napping can a person handle? Like I mentioned before, I mostly felt 'a little yucky', similar to having morning sickness. So, I wanted company—someone to 'just chat with'. Somebody to 'go have lunch with' or go

shopping with. Sure, I might tire out fairly quickly, but I

still wanted a life. I still wanted to live.

I quickly learned that most people do not know how

to respond to someone with a life-threatening illness. They

don't know what to say to them--so they generally just don't

say anything. They go on with their own lives (as they

should), but they tend to not think about what the ill person

might be thinking. In many cases, they may be thinking

they are doing the right thing, by 'giving them time to rest'.

Yes, a cancer patient needs extra rest; however, they

also need to feel like life is still going on. I wanted to share

what was happening to me, but most importantly, I wanted

to feel some normalcy in my life. It was important to spend

time with my friends like before I was sick. To help a sick

friend – keep being a friend – and spend time with your

friend. Doing 'special things' like providing food, cleaning their house, and collecting donations for extra

expenses will be appreciated, but remember to give them

some normalcy. Stop by, 'just to say hi'. Offer to go to

lunch with them, or go shopping. If they are too tired, they

will tell you, but don't wait for them to ask you to be there--

they may not...


**Changing Insurance and Oncologist - a New Experience**

After the six months on OHP, it was coming up for

renewal again, and Jon had been changed to a permanent

employee, so we no longer qualified. When the change

occurred, we had to switch to an HMO insurance to avoid

having a 'cap' placed on any charges for the cancer

treatments. My oncologist warned me that I needed to be

proactive in my care, because sometimes HMO's will do as

little as they think necessary.

At my first appointment with the new oncologist, he asked me if my previous oncologist, Dr. N had ever mentioned doing a stronger dosage for a shorter time (four months instead of six months). I told him no, but when I went back to see Dr. N for one more appointment, I asked him about it. His response was that if he had given me a stronger dosage, I would have ended up hospitalized because even at the original dosage, it was too strong for my body to handle. He had decreased it and added the three daily shots to bring my white cells back up. By adjusting my treatments and adding the three daily injections, I never had to have my treatments delayed in order to wait for my blood counts to come up again.

## Another Support Group

After having to switch insurances, I decided to try out the HMO support group. I was surprised to find out that

I had to pay a co-pay to attend their support group--

I had never heard of a support group where you had to pay

a co-pay to attend, but I decided to visit them anyway.

When I arrived, I entered the room where everyone

was seated in a circle of chairs, with maybe a dozen people

there. Soon after I sat down, a Vietnamese woman arrived,

accompanied by her husband. She did not speak a lot of

English, so they were hoping he could stay to help

translate, but the group leader told them the group was only

for women with breast cancer and he could not stay.

Reluctantly, she sat down next to me and he left.

As the group started, everyone was encouraged to

share what they were experiencing, how long since their

diagnosis and how things were going for them. While some

of the women shared, the Vietnamese lady kept saying

quietly, "I'm so scared--I'm so scared", yet no one seemed

to be hearing her besides me. Finally, I spoke up and said,

"She says she is very scared". So, the woman leading the group began asking her questions. The Vietnamese woman had been diagnosed with breast cancer several years before, and gone through treatments successfully, but now it had returned and was in her brain. She said she was filled with such a fear that she was unable to do normal daily things such as washing dishes. She was encouraged to share her feelings, but never really given an answer of how to help relieve her fears.

At the end of the group, the leader of the group, dimmed the lights and told everyone to close their eyes and think of a peaceful place. "BONG!" She had hit some sort of instrument... "Now think of a colored light, what ever color you want it to be..." She continued with a new age type of imagery, including making the "BONG" sound. As she continued, I imagined a nice warm beach and the light I imagined was God, but I quickly decided this group was

not for me and would be the last time I would visit.
Not only was I in disagreement about their new age theme,
I was not interested in paying to hear it.

## Meeting a New Friend

After the end of this group, I went to the
Vietnamese lady and spoke to her privately. I believe that it
was for this woman that God had me visit the group. I told
her that if she was interested, I attended another cancer
support group at a church that was for cancer patients of all
types of cancer, AND their support persons--her husband
could come with her. I told her that I realized she may be
from a different religion, but the people in this group were
from many different churches and beliefs.

I also shared with her a technique that I had found
helpful. I told her that whenever she felt scared, she should
stop and write out her feelings. I told her that I wrote those

feelings to God, but she could write them however she wanted, acknowledging her fears. Write down everything she was feeling and why she thought she was feeling that way. Then, give the paper to God (or who ever she believed in) by either tearing it up, or burning it. That way she was saying "Yes, I feel scared, but God, I'm giving those fears to you!" She thanked me for sharing and took the paper where I wrote down the name and dates for the church support group.

She did not arrive the next week at the church support group, but I shared my experience at that group and asked for prayers for her. The following week, she arrived with her husband and two children (the church provided daycare for participants in their groups). She said that she had been writing down her fears, like I had told her and then tore them up and that it had helped her. They came to a couple of our sessions, but they lived a bit of a distance from the church, and it meant a late night for their

young children.

The last time I saw them at our group, her

treatments seemed to be helping and she was doing better.

A few months later, our group leader received a call from

the husband, saying she had taken a sudden turn for the

worse and had died--he invited us to attend her funeral

service.

Some might say, "Well, she died--what help were

you?" Well, I believe that God put me in a place to meet

her and share God's love with her. This was to help her

proceed in the rest of the life she had remaining and build a

closer relationship with her children while she was there.

Sometimes we don't know why certain people arrive in our

paths, but we must learn to share when the opportunity

presents itself. Did this woman give her life to Christ? I

will never know, but if I was able to help give her some peace in her life, it was all worthwhile.

**One Bottle or Two - A Shortened Chemo?**

When I went into the new clinic for my last cycle of treatments, I discovered that they had a row of curtained cubicles, each with a hospital bed and the necessary supplies for connecting the patients with their IV chemo drugs. It somewhat reminded me of a production line--the nurses just went from one patient to the next, performing the next action. Heaven forbid, you would allow them to have conversations with each other. The nurse came in and 'plugged me in' to the IV drugs via my port; however, instead of the four hour treatments that I had been receiving, they did it in only two hours. I was surprised by this, but did not really think much about it--UNTIL later that night, when I began to feel increasingly sick. The next week when I went back to have blood work done to

see if my numbers were high enough for the next treatment,

I told my new oncologist that I had been receiving my

treatments in four hour sessions previously, and they had

done it in two hours--and I felt sicker! Could they please

do it in four hours? His response was "Sure, just tell the

nurse."

The next treatment--my FINAL treatment--I told the

nurse I wanted her to do it in four hours instead of two. Her

response was, "You want me to use two bags of glucose?"

I told her, "No, I just want you to slow it down. You gave it

to me last week in two hours and I got sicker, so I would

like to receive it in four hours, like I had received it from

my previous oncologist".

Two hours later, I was finished. I was thinking, oh

well, it is the last one; I'm not going to complain. Twenty

four hours later, when I found myself hovering over the

'Royal Throne', I wished that I had let everyone know. I was vomiting and my blood counts dropped so low, that if they would have dropped any further, I would have been hospitalized and given a blood transfusion. This was the ONLY time that I got sick enough from chemo to vomit!

I was down to zero immunity because the nurses could not figure out how to listen to my requests and do the treatment in a different way than they had been doing it. After all, they would not be able to do as many treatments for other patients if they slowed things down for me...

What this demonstrated to me was, if they would just slow the drip down, and allow it to take longer, my body would respond so much better, and would have less unpleasant side effects. Some of the chemo drugs are very toxic, and people have DIED from chemo. While administering the drugs quickly might be more efficient for the medical staff, it could make it worse on the

patient and possibly turn the treatment into a life

threatening situation. Why should the patient be put at

unnecessary risk, in order to save time for the medical

staff? Medical staff needs to learn to listen to the patient

instead of just following protocol.


**Summer, 1995--Connecting the Dots**

Chemo was finished, now it was time for the second

part of my treatments--radiation. In my opinion, radiation

was a piece of cake--it took longer to 'set me up' then to do

the actual treatment. But first came the preparation.

When I went in to prepare for the radiation series, I

realized that modesty was going to be a thing of the past.

While lying on a treatment table with nothing but my

underwear (no bra), they lined me up with laser beams and

marked me with several small tattoo dots. They then took a

Polaroid picture, so they could get the correct alignment for each treatment. Each time I would come back for my treatment, there on a clip on the wall—anyone walking by could see-- was the Polaroid picture of me, in all my glory! Truly a strange and awkward feeling…I still wonder what happened to that picture….

A little side-story: Those tattoo dots were just as permanent as a normal tattoo. Many years later when we were on a cruise, they played a game where they called out different things and the first team to send someone up with the called out item got points. They called out Tattoo, so I ran up and said, "See? I have a radiation dot tattoo?" And we got the points! LOL

Anyway, each day, five days a week, I went in for my radiation treatment. As I mentioned before, this was a very easy part of my treatments; however, I also have a sister-in-law for whom that was not the case. She had an

allergic reaction to radiation and ended up badly
burned, and her skin became very leathery. They had to
stop her radiation because her skin couldn't handle it.
Fortunately for most of us, that is a fairly rare reaction. I
got a slight redness, like a mild sunburn, and I was given
doctor's samples of Aquafor. I began using this gel several
times a day, BEFORE my skin began to burn and continued
through-out the six weeks of treatment. I think that
keeping the skin well hydrated is a key for reducing
reactions.

During this time, a friend taught me how to make
some beautiful 'glittery' shirts. I would find prints I liked
and 'gluc' it to the fabric of the shirt (T shirt or sweatshirt)
with an iron on webbing. Then, outline the edges in liquid
paint, followed by a sprinkle of glitter. These were
beautiful and we sold them at craft bazaars to make some
extra money. Frequently, I had been working on these

shirts before I went in for my treatments, and the glitter ended up everywhere. My radiation techs--and yes, they all seemed to be male--began to tease me about my 'sparkling personality'.

Another bit of awkward humor was as they lined me up for each treatment, they would make comments like, "That looks good..."  I remember thinking "Why thank you very much for thinking my breasts looked good!" *Remember, my radiation techs were ALL males...*

**A New Form of A/C**

In July, our denomination always held "Old Fashioned Camp Meeting" in Brooks, Oregon. My parents, siblings, and family had traditionally 'camped out together' at the church campgrounds, attending the daily services. I had finished my chemo treatments by then, and I had begun my daily radiation treatments. I decided to commute to the radiation treatments from Brooks to Portland,

Oregon--about a 45 minute drive each way. We were

having triple digit weather, which is unusual for our area of

Oregon, and the air-conditioning in our vehicle was not

working. With the heat, I had to drive with the windows

down, but that tangled my wig, so I was trying to not roll

them down very far. Finally, I decided, "Who cares? The

people on this freeway don't know me, and I don't care!" I

pulled off my wig, and laid it on the seat next to me and

rolled the windows down and drove freely! Of course, as

soon as I got off the freeway, I put the wig back on...

Later, while at the campground, I was feeling

sweaty under the wig, so I decided to go into the restroom

and get a cool damp paper towel to wipe off the top of my

head--it felt so good! I decided to place it back on my head,

and put the wig on over top of it and whenever I began to

feel warm again, I would pat the top of my head!

Hey, it worked!

During this time, Jon would jokingly say, "Hey! This is one time, when I have more hair than my wife!" And I would reply, "Yes, but mine will grow back and yours won't". We found the humor, wherever we could at that time.

## My "New Short Hairstyle"

When my hair started growing back, I was slow to gain enough courage to show it in public and continued wearing a wig or head wrap for a while. When I eventually stopped covering my head, my hair was still very short, but it was very curly. It curled around my fingers and I loved it! I had been attending a BC Support group, and there was a woman who had begun her treatments just before I did and her hair was looking similar to mine. She told us that one day, someone had asked her who her hair stylist

was and she replied "God!" I was disappointed that my hair

did not come back reddish, so, yes, I decided to try dying it,

and was quite happy with the results. I recently heard that

they now advise you to wait at least 6 months before dying

or 'perming' your hair--oh well. It worked for me with no

unwanted side effects...

I was sad that after the first time I had my haircut,

all the curls went away, and I also felt the stylist cut it too

short.

*Note to hairstylists cutting someone's hair for the*

*first time or two after losing their hair: Lean on the longer*

*side--after having NO hair, most women want to keep as*

*much length as possible to begin with--even if it means you*

*have to keep cutting "a little" more, your customer will*

*appreciate your concerns of her feelings.*

**Hormone Therapy**

The third part of my treatments was five years of hormone therapy with Tamoxifen. At first, I was uncertain about taking it because of some of the possible side effects. Just before I was supposed to start taking it, I went to a breast Cancer Survivor Event. At that event, I was able to ask questions of a doctor, who assured me that I did not have to be very concerned about the side effects. This regimen only involved taking a pill daily for five years. It hardly seemed like a treatment; however, I later found out that it was a very effective treatment.

A friend of mine, the leader of our Christian Support Group, had breast cancer years before me, and had received a mastectomy. She had no further treatments, but she developed a reoccurrence and they began giving her Tamoxifen, which was shrinking her tumor. Unfortunately for her, the cancer had spread to her bones and later took her life, but it proved to me that Tamoxifen really does work.

## Numbness and Lymphedema

One thing that my doctors never seemed to mention was how long the numbness would last in the arm where I had surgery. When they remove lymph nodes in the armpit, nerves are also cut, and the numbness from that can last for a significant amount of time--sometimes years. Generally, people tend to think that if something is numb, there is no pain--not true. There is an ongoing tingling that persists for some time and can be quite bothersome.

Also, since lymph nodes may be removed, and then later, radiation can kill even more lymph nodes, patients can develop Lymphedema. This is a swelling of the arm, because you no longer have the lymph nodes which drain off excess fluids. The effects of the condition can be anywhere from nonexistent to quite extensive. In my case, it was not really a problem at first.

As time went by, I started experiencing some swelling and was referred to a specialist to teach me (and Jon) how to do manual lymph drainage massage. We were also taught how to wrap my arm with four different wraps-- similar to those used for a sprain--with progressively higher amount of compression. I was instructed to do this 'wrap' which started at the fingers and went up to the armpit. This was done after the massage and then I was instructed to do some arm exercises with the wrap on.

Since the wrap went from fingertips to armpit, trying to do exercise with this on was not an easy task. I was also supposed to wear it to bed--which was NOT particularly comfortable. Since it was still summer and wearing the wrap made it feel even hotter, I eventually went longer times without putting it on, with the logic that, "mine isn't that bad". That was true; however, in the past year or so, I have had more swelling and my range of motion has become restricted. Yes, I need to go back--I can't even remember how to do the wraps now...

## My Happy & Cheerful Attitude

Many of my friends commented on my 'happy attitude' during this time. My response was that God had foretold us of his care and control, and I was trusting what He told us. I believed that God wanted us to look for the positive, while going through the negative and sometimes we even found some humor along the way. These are the things that gct us through the tough times   when we learn to lean and become 'overcomers' with God's help. I truly do not know how people without faith in God could make it through such difficult times.

I also believe that being depressed does nothing to improve our odds, and in fact, the opposite is true. Statistics have shown that those with a belief system and a positive outlook on life generally have a longer survival rate, and I chose that path for myself.

At one point, one of our teenage daughter's got upset with me about something, and said, "There you go again--bragging about having cancer!" Yes, her comment hurt to the core; however, I believe that I did not 'brag about having cancer", but I always tried to give glory to God, for being with me through my journey.

I share that to say that many times people may take our 'happy and cheerful attitude' in a wrong way. Maybe they don't understand that our happiness and cheerfulness comes from God, as we put our trust in Him. We should all remember what the Bible tells us about this in Proverbs 17:22. "A joyful heart is good medicine, but a crushed spirit dries up the bones."

## The Scare of Mammograms as a Survivor

Once you have had breast cancer, every follow-up mammogram is met with nerves a little on edge… Is this going to be bad news--am I going to be one of the 5% to have a reoccurrence? As the years go by, it gets a little easier, but it is always in the back of your mind.

Before I began traveling with Jon, I went in for a routine yearly mammogram, and was pleased to have another year behind me. Then it happened--I got a call-back. They saw something suspicious. I needed to return for them to take a second look. My heart dropped to the bottom of my stomach.

Suddenly, our future plans flashed before my eyes. What if this is IT? What happens to the travel plans we had been looking forward to? Was I going to have to go through this all again? Was Jon going to need to tell his manager that he couldn't take the new position? I was so nervous!

Fortunately, they were kind enough to get me scheduled quickly, but Jon had meetings he needed to attend and couldn't go with me. I was in my car returning from a quick errand before heading to the hospital for my follow-up mammogram, when I began listening to a song playing on our Christian radio channel.

This song had probably played on the radio hundreds of times, but this was the first time I REALLY heard the song. The song was called "They Don't Understand" by Brown Sawyer. The song talks about people going through hard times as others are getting frustrated with them, because "They Don't Understand". In my situation, it was not that anyone was getting frustrated with me and just didn't understand--it was that

nobody else knew what was going on at that very moment.

I still didn't know what the outcome would be, but I

knew that whatever the outcome, I was in God's hands and

He would carry me through. I amazed myself at how calm

I felt as I walked into the room to have that second X-ray.

The woman explained that if there was anything

questionable on the X-rays, they would then do an

ultrasound. She placed my breast into the 'smashing

machine' and stepped out to "see if she got a good look".

When she returned, she said "I don't see anything!" She

explained that sometimes it is 'just a shadow', but especially

with someone who has previously had cancer, they want to

be careful and make sure they got the best view they can

get. She told me I could go home, and unless the radiologist

saw something she didn't see, that it was 'good to go until

next year'.

Whew!  Good for another year--what beautiful words.

**When Breast Cancer Kills**

A dear friend of ours, the wife of a former pastor, was diagnosed with stage 4 cancer a few years ago. This brought me to a point of thinking once again about my own breast cancer journey and how wonderful that God had brought me through it; however, my dear friend Bobbi was dying from it.  This wonderful woman of God whose faith and determination to give God all the glory for every difficult thing in her life, was dying of the illness that I had fought and conquered.

Bobbie was a woman whom I had highly admired as did many other people who knew her.  How was it that God could take such a wonderful woman of God, yet allow me 20 more years after diagnosis? I have also known others

who have died as well, such as my aunts, the
Vietnamese lady I met in the support group, and my
Christian support group leader.

But this was a woman who trusted God and shared with
anyone and everyone who would listen to her.

God spoke to my heart. I felt that He assured me
that everyone has goals and things that God wants them to
accomplish. When they have accomplished those things,
then it is their time to die. We don't know when that time
is, and there are many things in this life that we may find
difficult to understand, but God makes His plan known to
us when we are in glory with Him.


## My Writing

Around the same time that I was questioning God
about my friend, I found out that another dear friend of

mine had published her first book--at age 88. I had always thought about

writing--I had enjoyed taking creative writing in high school, and many family and friends had said to me, "Vicki, you have experienced so many varied things in your life--you should write a book.

Many times I thought about their suggestion that I write a book--I had written journals and blogs and even a few book reviews, but I just didn't know what I should write about. Then a child within my family went through a horrible event in her life. I had previously read a novel about an adult who had gone through a similar event as a young girl and how it had later affected her life as an adult. I thought--hmm--maybe there is a novel for young girls that have gone through a similar situation which could help this family member; however, when I checked, I found no such books. My next thought was, "hmm--God, are you telling me this is what I should write?", and I felt God's answer was yes.

Yes, my writing has gotten temporarily sidetracked, by other writing (such as this memoir), but the story for young girls is still in progress and I fully intend to finish it when God tells me the time is right.

## Change in Job Roles--Sept. 2008

In 2008, Jon had the opportunity to change job roles at his company and it was going to mean a LOT of travel. I was going to 'follow him around the world' while his company reimbursed my airfare when the trips were international. My first trip with him was four weeks in Paris and then we took the High-Speed train through the Chunnel (the tunnel under the English Channel) to London. We spent the night in London before going to a small town south of London named Horsham for four weeks. Then, we flew to Madrid for another four weeks--meaning we did not go home for three months!  It was a long time away from home, but it was our first time ever for foreign travel, so we thoroughly enjoyed it.

This was the beginning of our life with a crazy travel schedule. Our typical schedule is to have a week in between engagements, with four weeks away from home. In the past six years, we have traveled to more than 20 different countries, most of which included a four week stay. When the company reimburses the airfare, additional taxes are taken from Jon's pay. Nevertheless, most of the travel costs are airfare, hotel and food. We can share many of our meals, and we have 'status' with some hotel chains, so usually, there is no extra charge for me at the hotels. This means we can do what many people hope to do when they retire – and that is to travel the world. Sometimes we will be watching a game show, and see a prize like a 'week in Paris' valued at several thousand dollars, and we smile, thinking, 'we've done that'—more than once!

We do not get to see our grandchildren as much as we might like, but we are making a lifetime of memories. In 2007, we thought we might do some travel, and we applied for passports. Now, in 2014, we had to order 'extra pages' for our passports so we would have room for more 'visa' stamps. To be able to travel this much continues to be an incredible blessing, and we thank God for his protection and promises. It is almost hard to believe how quickly the time has gone by—even more now where we change cities every month.

### A Hope and A Future

Jon's vision of what 'looked like an X-ray' was a shadow of the valley of death. But God was faithful— before we even knew there was a problem, he promised a way through. We also knew that we would have to go THROUGH the valley, and there would be no shortcuts. Through that ordeal, we met wonderful people and had the opportunity to share God's goodness.

As I look back on the 20 years since my diagnosis, I am especially thankful for all of those who stood with me during the hard times. I hope everyone who reads this will accept our thanks for all of the help and prayers. We will continue to pray for each of you, that God will bless each of you as richly as he has blessed us.

**Final Thoughts:**

This edition was prepared prior to Vicki's 20th anniversary celebration. In the final version, we will be including reference material which we hope will help those that are facing life-changing illness. The topics we plan to include are:

How to prepare for doctor appointments

How to find the things you need (wigs, head wraps, etc.)

Thoughts and advice for the spouse

Thoughts and advice for helping the children

What to look for in a support group

Links for resources